I0091082

Intermittent Fasting for Women Over 50

How You Can Effortlessly Lose Weight, Balance Your Hormones and Increase Energy and Focus with Intermittent Fasting

Rebekah Addams

© **Copyright 2020 – Rebekah Addams All rights reserved.**

The content contained within this book may not be reproduced, duplicated or transmitted without direct written permission from the author or the publisher.

Under no circumstances will any blame or legal responsibility be held against the publisher, or author, for any damages, reparation, or monetary loss due to the information contained within this book, either directly or indirectly.

Legal Notice:

This book is copyright protected. It is only for personal use. You cannot amend, distribute, sell, use, quote or paraphrase any part, or the content within this book, without the consent of the author or publisher.

Disclaimer Notice:

Please note the information contained within this

document is for educational and entertainment purposes only. All effort has been executed to present accurate, up to date, reliable, complete information. No warranties of any kind are declared or implied. Readers acknowledge that the author is not engaged in the rendering of legal, financial, medical or professional advice. The content within this book has been derived from various sources. Please consult a licensed professional before attempting any techniques outlined in this book.

By reading this document, the reader agrees that under no circumstances is the author responsible for any losses, direct or indirect, that are incurred as a result of the use of the information contained within this document, including, but not limited to, errors, omissions, or inaccuracies.

Table of Contents

Intermittent Fasting Cheat Sheet

Before we get started, I wanted to first of all say thank you for choosing this book to help get you started in the world of intermittent fasting. It is without a doubt the most sustainable and efficient way to get into shape, detox your body and live a healthy lifestyle.

If you would like extra support from myself, I would love for you to join my private Facebook group, where you can speak to me directly ask any questions you might have on how to apply fasting to you specifically.

I am always happy to help and and it will give you a chance to mix with other people on the same path as you.

Just search for **Intermittent Fasting, Fuel the Brain, Lose the Fat** on Facebook, request to join, answer the 3 questions and I'll accept you straight away.

I would also like to give you my intermittent fasting cheat sheet which will be a valuable tool in ensuring your on the right track from the very start. It will give you a check list of the most important aspects of fasting to look out for, I want you to get the most out of this new lifestyle and prevent any of the common mistakes that a lot of newbies make initially.

Just go to **www.thefastingfacts.com** and I will send to straight to your email.

Introduction

Being fit and healthy and losing weight is fast becoming an unattainable goal, a deceptive, elusive mirage. People run from one diet plan to another, from one exercise regimen to another, all in the name of trying to stay fit. Who wouldn't want to be healthy, keep diseases at bay, and enjoy a long happy life? But what these strenuous diets give you are nothing but temporary weight loss and additional stress. Stress in the form of extensive meal planning and giving up your favorite foods along with additional costs of maintaining such diets and hitting the gym regularly. No wonder then that many of us who try these diets and regimens do not go past a few months at the most.

People get tired of the constant need to keep their food intake in check, monitor their calories, and make sure that they are burning enough of those calories through physical exercise. When you decide to follow a particular diet, you are excited, enthusiastic and looking forward to new changes in the beginning, but as time passes the enthusiasm fades and maintaining these changes becomes a chore. The biggest reason for this is that these changes are dietary changes and are not incorporated as a lifestyle change.

At the end of a failed diet plan we are back to square one, with the weight that we had lost back, along with a horde of other health problems that arise with the weight gain, needless to mention the challenges that increasing age presents us with. So, is being healthy and losing weight truly this difficult? Have we, with all our advanced scientific discoveries and inventions, still not come up with something that truly helps in the long run?

Have we discovered the root of all our health and weight issues? I believe we have. All this time, though our understanding of why we gain weight is good enough, our approach to shedding that said weight was entirely wrong. Through intermittent fasting we cannot just lose excess weight but also work toward staying healthy and fit. To all our weight gain issues and health problems because of it, intermittent fasting is the answer.

For women, weight gain is a real problem after marriage and motherhood. With all the hormones and body changes that a woman faces right from attaining puberty, marriage, pregnancy, childbirth, breastfeeding, to menopause, and post-menopausal changes, it is nothing short of a roller coaster ride. Women with their inherent strengths are great at handling all these changes and different life roles with ease. But, needless to say, this takes a toll on their bodies and by the time a woman is past the childbearing age and within the menopausal or post-menopausal stage, her body is not how it was in her youth anymore.

If a woman wishes to lose weight and take charge of her body and health once again after the age of 50, these diet plans and extensive exercises would be of no help at all. These will become more and more difficult to stick to and follow through. Adding to this, physical exercises will become increasingly daunting to perform at this age. So how should women work to maintain their health and reduce unwanted weight? Again, intermittent fasting is the most appropriate and veracious method to counter these issues.

Intermittent fasting helps you to reduce weight and keep diseases at bay, along with helping you become more productive, saving your time and efforts on meal planning and preparation, saves your money investments, and gives you greater mental clarity and sharpness. Several diet studies and research have lead scientists to conclude that intermittent fasting is indeed extremely effective with little to no negatives once it is adopted as a lifestyle by a person. Intermittent fasting is nothing new to mankind. It has its roots in several major religions worldwide that include fasting as a religious ritual. Apart from this, fasting also has strong relevant support in the works of famous scholars of the past such as Plato, Socrates, and the like.

The biggest advantage to intermittent fasting is that your focus here is not on what you eat but rather on when you eat it. The whole system works around scheduling your eating habits rather than monitoring what you are eating. There are no regrets of missing out on favorite foods or chances of guilty pleasures. It is a game of patience and consistency that lets extended periods of fasting do the job, instead of restricted calorie intake or physical exertions.

This is not to say that any and all types of food are welcome, but rather to say that extensive critical monitoring is not required. Your focus should be to eat healthy food without overindulgence in junk and naturally unhealthy foods. It is also important to note that intermittent fasting helps you cleanse your body of toxins and other harmful substances. Therefore, it is of little sense to fill your body with junk when all you wish to do is cleanse your body of it through intermittent fasting. Afterall, this cleansing is what helps you stay healthy and avoid diseases of almost any and every kind.

There is hardly a person out there who wishes to shed the extra pounds who hasn't dabbled in one theory of weight loss or the other. The fact that you are reading this book is a testament to your commitment to staying healthy and fit. It is important therefore that you gather all the knowledge there is to know about intermittent fasting, bundle up your resources and prepare yourself before you take the plunge.

Intermittent fasting is all about staying constant and committed. Around the world, and in America specifically, obesity and unwanted weight gain has become a huge problem. It is high time that we take measures to ensure we and those around us are healthy and stay away from problems of excessive weight loss. Adopt and embrace intermittent fasting as your way of life and I can assure you that you shall see a marked difference in your body weight, your general wellbeing, and your overall health. It is far easier to cross a small hurdle and maintain your health with constancy than scaling a huge wall of mental and physical health transformation when things get tough. And eventually things will get tough if proper care is not given to your body and health beforehand and if no efforts are made at all to maintain fitness.

Give yourself and your body the love and attention it deserves by taking deliberate measures to follow intermittent fasting. Though it will be difficult in the beginning, as time goes on and you stick to following it with commitment, you will come to love your body and the changes that intermittent fasting has brought about within you.

Chapter 1: What Is Intermittent Fasting?

Now that we have introduced the concept of intermittent fasting, let's try to understand in depth what it truly means and how it really works. Intermittent fasting is nothing but fasting for extended periods of time and eating only within an allowed window of time. So, what does fasting do and how does it help you lose weight?

Feeding and Fasting

Our body is continuously in one of two states, which are the feeding or fasting states. When we eat a meal, our body is in the feeding state and it remains in this state for the next 4 to 5 hours. We do not feel hungry in this state. After about 6 to 8 hours comes the post feeding state or the intermediate state, where we may or may not feel hungry, and the body uses our most recent meal to gather energy when needed for some action. After this comes the fasting stage, which lasts until we have another meal.

During this fasting stage, because we haven't taken a meal, and our body has already used the last meal to derive energy, it now turns to our stored energy reserves which are the fats in our body. This is the stage when fats get burned. In this stage we feel hungry and our body looks for food to use as fuel, but upon not finding any recent meal, because we haven't eaten, burns our fat stores. This is why fasting has been known to be such an important way to burn accumulated fats. But if we have provided our body with food, then it doesn't enter the fasting stage and no fat gets burned and our body resorts to our next meal for energy.

The Science Behind Intermittent Fasting

To understand how intermittent fasting works, it is important to understand what normally happens in our bodies with the food we eat. Whenever we take a meal, eat or even drink something, our body releases a hormone called insulin. Insulin is widely popular as a medicine given to diabetics but not much thought is given to it as to the why and the how of it.

This insulin released at the time of consumption of food acts as the monitor of our blood glucose levels. Insulin takes care of the amount of glucose we need immediately as energy for our actions. It decides how much of this glucose should be converted to glycogen, which is nothing but an easily available energy source, and how much of it should be stored as fat for later use. This is the reason why insulin is also known as a fat-storing hormone. Some diabetics are unable to have this glucose monitor in their blood and hence need external insulin injections to handle their blood glucose levels.

If you are constantly or regularly eating, then your body is regularly releasing insulin. This leads to more and more storage of energy in the form of fats. Your body has no chance to reach your already present fat reserves to burn them for energy;

instead it is adding to them constantly. So, one important thing to keep in mind is to keep your insulin levels in check, and this can be easily done through proper scheduling of your meals.

Two other important hormones that regulate our hunger and appetite are ghrelin and leptin. Ghrelin is known as the hunger hormone as this is the hormone responsible for causing us hunger and pushing us to eat more. If your regular eating schedule involves three meals a day, then your body secretes the ghrelin hormone at your three mealtimes to signal it is time to eat. Ghrelin release does not necessarily mean your body is in need of food, it simply means it is your regular eating time and your body is reminding you to eat. You can regulate ghrelin levels by intermittent fasting so that your body gets adjusted to your new eating schedules.

Leptin is another important hormone that helps regulate your food intake. It is also called the satiety hormone, because it signals that you have had enough food and hints you to stop eating. It helps you feel full and satisfied. The higher the leptin levels the less likely you are to eat food. Naturally, since birth, we are wired to have a balance of both ghrelin and leptin levels, but with our ever changing lifestyles and unhealthy food practices, that causes this inherent balance to be disturbed and these hormone levels swing either way, causing us to put on more weight through unregulated eating habits.

You see the best demonstration of the working of these hormones in infants and also in toddlers to some extent. Children in these age groups have their own minds of when they would like to eat and how much. This is their hormones talking and they are often doing a better job than us to keep our food intake in check. Most often we see parents struggling to feed their toddlers, running around the house or the backyard trying to get a few bites in. The thing is, a toddler generally doesn't eat when they are full. Their leptin tells them they have had enough, and they refuse to eat more. We, as concerned parents, sometimes force them to eat. Here begins the imbalance of these hormones.

Leptin no longer functions properly, because we seem to eat even when it is signaling us not to. Right from that age, we begin to tell our brains we eat at certain times, or because we have food on hand, or we have something before us that we absolutely cannot pass up. This messes up with the hormone signals. We are not eating like we used to in the infant to toddler age, when we are hungry; instead we eat because it is our supposed mealtime, even if we are not feeling the need. All the three hormones, insulin, ghrelin, and leptin, are now in quite an imbalanced state, leading us to feel hungry all the time, causing us to eat all the time, thereby increasing our fat storage.

Six Meals A Day - The Wrong Approach

In most diets, the most popular phenomenon is to divide your whole food intake per day into six or more small portions. These meals are taken throughout the day with a gap of a few hours in between. It has been a popular belief for quite some time now that doing so helps your metabolism and helps reduce weight because you aren't feeding on large quantities at once. Instead, what this truly does is keeps your insulin levels constantly high. What this does in turn is convert all the digested sugars into fats.

Naturally in a single day, you wouldn't require all the energy that even six small meals could give you. So, the sugar monitor in your blood, insulin, directs all the unused sugars to be turned into fat and stored for later. Doing this day in and day out, every day, simply increases your fat stores. We need to use up the already stored fat not add more to it. But that is exactly what eating several small meals in a day does. Only when we give time to our body to reduce its insulin levels in the blood, will it be able to access the stored fat and use that for energy. This is impossible when a constant food intake is going on. The time intervals between these small meals is too small to induce our bodies into accessing the stored fat, because it still has glucose from the most recent meal to make use of.

Therefore, contrary to popular belief, six or more small meals is in reality the wrong way to go about it. The need of the hour is to look for something that gives your body sufficient time to reach those stored fats and burn them, and intermittent fasting is ideal for just that!

Benefits of Intermittent Fasting for Women Over 50

Researchers have found that for older women who are either in the premenopausal or postmenopausal stages, around the age of 50, intermittent fasting is just as beneficial as for younger people. Though there are a few medical and physical conditions that will have to be satisfied for one to take up intermittent fasting, and we shall see in later chapters what these are, it is extremely beneficial for several reasons.

Weight loss decreased levels of insulin and increased HGH levels, better metabolism, and better muscle and bone health are just a few of the many benefits of intermittent fasting at this age. Increased HGH levels cause our bodies to burn excess fats and encourage muscle growth. Another chemical, called the noradrenaline is also released by our bodies to help burn fat cells for fuel when in a fasting stage. Belly fat is a constant worry for most women beyond menopause, and intermittent fasting is great at burning and reducing belly fat. Also, better bone health has always been a much sought after requirement for older women around the world, and intermittent fasting is a step in the right direction to ensure your bone and muscle health improves.

Autophagy

Autophagy is when our body destroys and eliminates cells that are no longer needed. It is a cleansing mechanism wherein our body recognizes damaged, useless, or toxic cells and eliminates them. It is a self-cleansing method employed by our bodies and is often triggered in the fasting stage.

When we sleep at night, the first part of the night is dedicated to correcting our bodies physical damages and addressing its physiological needs. Any repair or restoration of cells and tissues that is needed to be done is done in this first part of the night. The next half of the night is dedicated to correction of mental issues or problems. Things that cause us stress and worry are supposedly addressed in this period, when we are in a deep sleep. This is the reason why when we are stressed, we often find ourselves awake and unable to go back to sleep in the middle of the night, because our body is urging us to solve or resolve whatever stress we are going through.

This first part of the night includes the autophagy mechanism and this cleansing process can also be duplicated during the daytime with the help of fasting. Fasting helps you get rid of toxins and harmful substances, and autophagy is a huge part of this process. We do not want unwanted damaged cells or dysfunctional cells using up our valuable energy resources, and so these are destroyed and eliminated through autophagy. This cleansing process gives us vitality bringing us a healthier and energetic working system. Our cells and tissues are healthier leading us to feel healthy and rejuvenated in return.

Drawbacks of Intermittent Fasting for Women Over 50

Intermittent fasting has a few drawbacks, especially in the beginning stages, when a person is still getting accustomed to retimed eating schedules. These drawbacks are few. For women, who can and cannot apply intermittent fasting schedules is a matter of deciding based on one's medical and physical conditions, which we shall look at later on in the book. But once a woman has decided and begun fasting, it is only a matter of adjusting and adapting oneself to the new eating patterns. Whatever disadvantages or drawbacks arise due to intermittent fasting, all stem from this adjustment stage.

Severe hunger pangs, lightheadedness, dizziness, dehydration, headaches, and muscle weakness are some of the problems that people normally face due to intermittent fasting schedules, and these too are restricted to the adapting or adjusting stage. One rare drawback of the fasting system is infertility. But this is hardly an issue after a couple of weeks of stopping the schedule and less so for women over 50 who are mostly beyond the child-bearing age.

Chapter 2: Intermittent Fasting and Medical Conditions

It is vital to know and understand how intermittent fasting affects various medical conditions and whether it improves or deteriorates the condition and how. Before we look at the effects of intermittent fasting on specific health conditions, let's look at who cannot do intermittent fasting.

When Should You Not Do Intermittent Fasting?

There are a few conditions for when intermittent fasting is not advisable.

Pregnant or Breastfeeding

It is highly discouraged to do intermittent fasting when a woman is either pregnant or breastfeeding. Both of these situations require a constant supply of balanced nutrients in the bloodstream and this is impossible to achieve through intermittent fasting. However balanced diets you consume in your eating periods will still fall short during the fasting window when the only available energy resources are the fats. This will not only be harmful to the baby but also to the mother, as all the available resources are put in use for meeting the baby's needs and this deprives the mother of much needed nutrients and energy resources.

Type 1 Diabetics

Type 1 diabetics are another group of people who are widely discouraged from taking part in any form of fasting schedules. This is because, in Type 1 diabetes a person is unable to produce any insulin. This makes the blood glucose levels go high because the body needs insulin to make use of blood glucose and it is absent in these cases. Type 1 diabetics are unequivocally discouraged from intermittent fasting as it is highly risky and dangerous. Since intermittent fasting primarily brings insulin levels down, therefore we wouldn't want to bring down its levels when they are already low or rather completely lacking in the bloodstream. It is therefore highly discouraged and Type 1 diabetics are rightly advised to stay away from intermittent fasting or any fasting schedules for that matter. It is better to be safe than to be sorry.

Eating Disorders and Underweight

People who have eating disorders of any kind, such as anorexia or bulimia, are discouraged from taking part in intermittent fasting. It is highly inadvisable to put your body through strenuous fasting routines when it is already suffering from the effects of disorderly eating habits. Also, people who are already underweight, which means their body weights fall below the ideal weight for their age and height are also discouraged from doing intermittent fasting. Not only would it not be ideal, but it would be highly inappropriate and unnecessary to coerce your body into even more restrictive eating habits. If you have a history of eating disorders, fasting of any sort is highly discouraged, as it can be a trigger to prior destructive patterns. There are better suited ways for you to regain and maintain your health, in this case.

Consulting Your Doctor

If you do not fall into any of these categories but are still doubtful of whether you can do intermittent fasting or not, it is always better to consult your doctor before you begin. Tell your doctor your wish to participate in intermittent fasting and place all your health concerns before them. Only when they give you the go ahead, is it proper for you to begin planning your fasts.

Type 2 Diabetes and Intermittent Fasting

Type 2 diabetics are the people who are insulin resistant. Insulin resistance is when your body is producing insulin, but you are unable to make use of it to monitor your blood glucose. To understand it better, there is another way of looking at it.

Imagine if you are used to eating non-stop round the clock. You are used to munching on snacks or any available food on the go. What this does is keep your insulin levels high all the time. After a certain period of time your body gets used to these elevated levels of insulin. This requires you to produce even more insulin after mealtimes, because your body has in a way, "stopped listening" to the normal levels. This goes on until your body is no longer able to make use of the insulin present in the bloodstream though you are able to produce it.

This is called insulin resistance. People with Type 2 diabetes have been known to benefit from monitored food intake and regular exercise. This is even more true in cases where intermittent fasting was applied. Type 2 diabetics were able to control their insulin levels and blood glucose levels with the help of intermittent fasting techniques. Obesity and unnatural weight gain are mostly common in people with Type 2 diabetes. And this is effectively handled and addressed by participating in intermittent fasting. If you are a Type 2 diabetic, talk with your doctor on what type of fasting would suit you. Work with your physician to know what mode of fasting would benefit you most keeping your diabetes and your other health and physical parameters in mind.

Cancer and Intermittent Fasting

Intermittent fasting has been known to be of several benefits to the human body, one of which is the prevention of cancer. Intermittent fasting works to help tackle several other health risks that are in turn factors for the development of cancer. Conditions like diabetes, obesity etc., are linked to rise in cancer cases. Intermittent fasting helps tackle these in turn helping protect us against cancer. Another important reason for seeing intermittent fasting as beneficial to cancer prevention and treatment could be because fasting helps regulate blood sugar, it triggers stem cells to produce more and more immune boosting cells and also tumor-killing cells. With the help of balanced nutritional intake, precursors to cancer are held in check by following an intermittent fasting schedule.

Studies on mice and other animals also showed how intermittent fasting could help produce better outcomes of chemotherapy in the treatment of cancer. Reduction of toxicity was another important observation after following intermittent fasting, which is valuable in cancer treatments.

Alzheimer's Disease and Intermittent Fasting

From research conducted by neuroscientists it has been concluded that fasting helps your brain get in control of neurodegenerative diseases such as Alzheimer's. Fasting has also been found to help improve memory and mood. This is mainly because fasting and intermittent fasting in particular, initiate the process of autophagy.

Autophagy has been found to be extremely important and beneficial in the treatment of neurological disorders like Alzheimer's and Parkinson's diseases. Fasting has been known to initiate macro autophagy in neurons in Alzheimer's patients, providing helpful relief and erasure of their symptoms.

Through research in animal models it was also observed that not only treatment but also prevention can occur through following intermittent fasting schedules. It is a known fact that intermittent fasting improves cognitive abilities, but it was also observed that intermittent fasting also helps against the deterioration of these cognitive abilities and improves memory. This is vital to prevent Alzheimer's and other neurodegenerative diseases like Parkinson's.

Heart Disease and Intermittent Fasting

Potential risk factors that might cause heart diseases can be effectively improved by following a fasting schedule. Intermittent fasting in particular, has been shown to have positive effects in terms of improving one's heart health. This can probably be related to how intermittent fasting causes one's fat reserves to be burned. This can cause your body to regulate your 'bad' cholesterol levels in turn helping you have a healthy heart. This can also be because people who practice intermittent fasting have better self-control. This self-control can help them make better eating choices. Not just what you eat but when you eat matters too. And intermittent fasting schedules help you monitor just that. Intermittent fasting reduces your chances of gaining unhealthy weight and developing diabetes, which are potential risk factors and known precursors to heart issues, thereby preventing heart problems.

Chapter 3: Losing Weight After 50

As much as it has been found to be easier to put on weight after 50, it is equally difficult to lose the same weight. Intermittent fasting can be highly beneficial in overcoming challenges to losing weight after the age of 50 which can otherwise become an unattainable goal through other means. There are a few health factors specific to women 50 years and older that can hinder efficient weight loss. Let's explore those next.

Metabolism

Before we begin to understand how metabolism differs after the age of 50, let's first understand what metabolism means. Metabolism is nothing but a collection of processes that occur inside a cell that help generate energy. This energy is vital to produce new compounds or carry out different actions. Metabolic rate is the amount of energy an organism, animal or human, uses per unit of time. This is measured when the organism is at rest or inactive and is known as the basal metabolic rate.

For women, their basal metabolic rate is known to decrease by about two to three percent every decade as they age. It is apparent therefore that a woman's basal metabolic rate will eventually fall as she ages, and it will be quite low when she is over 50 compared to when she was about 20 years of age. This is vital to consider seeing how metabolism is what drives us into food intake and calorie burning. This decrease in basal metabolism is what causes you to gain weight after a certain age.

Therefore, it is essential that you work toward improving your metabolism as you age and in turn keep your weight gain in check. It is also important to note that intermittent fasting increases our levels of HGH hormone which is vital for muscle repair and fat burning and which is naturally at a decline after the age of 50, as well. Therefore, practicing intermittent fasting can help you rev up your metabolism and also enhance your HGH production so that fat burn is at its efficient best while working with faster metabolism.

But it is also a known fact that when people eat less in the name of diet control and take in fewer calories, your body goes into protective mode and slows down your metabolic rate to cover the low caloric intake. This is also why lower metabolism makes losing weight difficult. After the age of 50, research has shown that both muscle mass and muscle strength decrease considerably each year. A woman may lose muscle mass up to 1 to 2 percent each year while losing muscle strength similarly. This is countered by the body by decreasing the basal metabolic rate, in short, the rate at which energy is normally used. This decreased metabolism again causes weight gain. All in all, metabolism, from whichever angle it is studied, seems to decrease after 50 causing weight gain issues in older women.

Injuries

As the years pass and we age, we accumulate a number of injuries through various unfortunate accidents. These injuries could be of any type, from bone fractures and joint dislocations to muscle tears and muscle sprains. Even if we aren't suffering from any immediate or apparent side effects of these injuries at present, still these injuries become a point of weakness in our bodies inhibiting active and agile movements. This becomes vital when we plan to exercise as normal exercise would then be difficult.

Even if there is no history of any kind of injuries, we might have simple muscle and joint weakness, causing sufficient pain which can again make exercise a huge chore. Muscle stiffness and joint pains can make it harder to perform even the most basic warm up exercises, for example. This is an expected change in older women and is seen to increase as the age increases. Some women have even complained of their older operation wounds and stitches flaring up with pain as they age. This again makes exercising difficult. This is why active exercise that can even be mildly strenuous is almost impossible for older women.

If you could once lift up weights, perform push-ups, work your abs with ease at a gym, all this become increasingly difficult after the age of 50. This is why women after 50 do not take losing weight as an achievable goal, and sometimes give up because the usual crucial requirement of exercise is out of reach for most women. This is not considering women who are physically active and are well habituated to exercising regularly. This is about those women who wish to shed their unhealthy weight and find it difficult to include an exercise regimen in their lives. This is why intermittent fasting is essential and most beneficial as it does not depend on physical movement of activity alone to counter weight gain.

Hormonal Changes and Menopause

Women undergo a horde of hormonal changes around, during, and after menopause. To understand these changes better let's understand what menopause truly is. A woman is born with all the eggs that they would release in their lifetime. These eggs are stored in the follicles in the ovaries. The ovaries release hormones such as estrogen and progesterone. As follicles decrease and the production of these two hormones decreases, the ovaries become increasingly less responsive to two more hormones that are related to reproductive activities, like luteinizing hormone (LH) and follicle stimulating hormone (FSH).

A woman's body undergoes three distinct stages with relation to menopause. Perimenopause, menopause, and post-menopause. Perimenopause is the stage before the menopause, beginning around eight to ten years before actual menopause begins. Menopause is when ovaries cease to release eggs and estrogen production slows (some is still produced by the adrenal glands).

When a woman goes without having her monthly periods for a period of one year it is termed as menopause. It is a normal natural phenomenon in aging women. Usually, menopause is normally seen in women aged 45 to 55 years of age. Post-menopause is the stage after the year long period-free stage. The usual menopausal symptoms of hot flashes, sudden night sweats or cold flashes, or vaginal dryness cease or diminish in this stage.

But the post-menopausal stage can bring about many different health issues such as diabetes, heart problems, and weight gain. These hormonal changes naturally make losing weight during these periods difficult. Extensive dietary restrictions, or strict exercise regimens are difficult to follow and not very effective for unaccustomed women for whom such measures are entirely new. This is again another reason why, for women of this age intermittent fasting is a wise course of action in order to counter unhealthy weight gain.

Diet Related Issues

With time and age, one's gut health deteriorates considerably. This is primarily due to poor food choices over the course of many years. After years of exposure to unhealthy or junk food, or food that is rich in complex fats, heavy carbs, and harsh spices, the stomach and intestinal lining take a hit. Imagine a motor or a machine that works at crushing or powdering hard substances. If all that is fed to this machine is hard stones and granite, over the course of some time, the machine would begin to deteriorate. Its blades might become blunt and it might considerably slow down. Compare this to a machine that has only been fed wood. Being softer and easier to crush than stones, these machines and its blades would naturally last longer than the previous one. This is very similar to what happens with our digestive tracts.

The more complex food we feed ourselves over time, the more tired our system gets as we age. It is therefore essential to keep our digestive system healthy by not taxing it too much. Combine this with weight gain and you have a tough one on your hands. Again, intermittent fasting can be of immense help. It improves your intestinal health by giving your body sufficient time to self-repair and replenish the lost tissues adequately between meals. This is a vital advantage in people with particularly sensitive and delicate gut health. Intermittent fasting will help these people strengthen their digestion and become confident of what they consume in their eating windows without fear of an upset stomach or any ill health.

Stress

For pre-menopausal and menopausal women, these stages can be stressful. A woman is already undergoing irregular periods, hot or cold flashes, and increased heart rate or palpitations. These along with increased hunger pangs, dehydration, heartburn, headaches and dizziness, from intermittent fasting can make this phase even more stressful. It is vital to take things slowly and easily during this period. A woman may become moodier and crankier due to the many physiological changes going on in her body and adding intermittent fasting to it without thought can make it more stressful.

If a woman undergoing menopause wishes to practice intermittent fasting it is extremely essential to start slow with one of the lighter versions of this fasting technique (that we'll talk about later). Being constantly under stress will make it more difficult for you to lose weight. As much as losing weight is a physiological phenomenon it is also a mental phenomenon that requires you to stay calm and in a happier state of mind.

It has been observed that people who gain unnatural amounts of weight or who are obese are in some way or the other stressed by something in their lives. Weight gain has been linked to feelings of abandonment, loneliness, and past or current abuse, which in turn gives rise to depression. Effective and thorough resolution of these feelings or addressing problems that give rise to such feelings can be an important first step in losing weight. Intermittent fasting does not demand any physical activity or exercise. It is good if you can squeeze it in your day to day routines. But what it does require is a positive frame of mind. Remove all negativity. Forgive and forget any past situations and scenarios that troubled you or people who caused you grief. Start your schedule with a fresh slate with a fresh frame of mind. Being stress free is extremely essential to long lasting weight loss.

Chapter 4: Types of Intermittent Fasting

There are several types of intermittent fasting techniques that one can choose to practice. They all differ based on the number of hours of fast time and number of meals in the day, and frequency of fasts or gap between fasts. They are important to know to decide what type of intermittent fasting would suit you best. For people who are just starting out and simply testing the waters, it is essential to start light. So, let's look at all the different types of intermittent fasting techniques that are in practice.

12/12 Method

This is a fairly easy method and is mostly adopted by beginners who are yet to get acclimatized to fasting. This method requires you to fast for 12 hours and have an open eating window of 12 hours. Again, how you adjust the hours of fasting and eating is entirely up to you as long as the hour ratio is maintained. Once a person has the feel of fasting through the 12/12 method they can gradually move onto more difficult or intense fasts.

14/10 Method

This is like a gradual step up from the 12/12 fasts. This method demands a fasting period of 14 hours with a ten-hour eating window. It is a great method to gradually ease oneself into more demanding fasting schedules such as the widely popular 16/8 method. But in comparison to the 16/8 method, this is known to be an extremely flexible method by how it balances the eating and fasting hours ideal for people who have physically demanding lifestyles and also those who wish for longer eating periods.

16/8 Method

This method is one of the most popular of all the intermittent fasting techniques. This requires you to fast for sixteen hours while having an eight-hour eating window. Many people opt to adjust their eating hours, so that their eating window coincides with the hours they need to be more active making their fasting hours align with their sleeping hours plus a few more. A night person would similarly delay their eating window to the night and extend their fast to the day. As long as the 16/8 hour ratio is maintained, a person is at liberty to adjust their eating and fasting hours as they wish.

20/4 Method

This is one step above the 16/8 Method. It requires an intense fast of twenty hours and has an open window of only four hours. People who are very well accustomed to intermittent fasting techniques over a course of at least a few weeks can look to adopt this method. This is a more demanding method and therefore requires that you take special care of what you consume in your eating window. High energy foods that can last for longer durations of time are ideal for these fasts. Make it an absolute must to stay entirely away from junk or wasteful filler food, that only fill you up with no nutrients instead cause you more harm. Make your food choices wisely ensuring to include healthy balanced choices in the four-hour window.

OMAD

This is another intense and tough regime to follow. Ideal for those who have been at it for quite some time now. OMAD stands for one meal a day. The person is free to choose which meal they would like to eat in a day, and they simply eat a meal at the same time the next day. This gives the person a fast of around 23 hours. That one meal must be nutritious and balanced so as to be able to sustain the person for the whole day. One who is following this extreme regimen is allowed one hour to partake a meal. They can eat anything in this hour as long as it is healthy and filling. The person is then allowed to take calorie-free beverages during the remaining 23 hours of fast. This is a rigorous type of intermittent fasting and is best suitable for seasoned practitioners.

5/2 Method

This is another rigorous method of fasting. It requires you to eat for five consecutive days while fasting for the remaining two consecutive days. This method doesn't require a complete or absolute fast for the two consecutive fasting days. Instead, the person is allowed to eat the minimum calorie requirement, around 25% of the caloric requirement, or about 500 to 600 calories in the two fasting days. The remaining five days are used to eat normally as the person is normally accustomed to eating. This presents a rigorous fast that requires a restricted diet of just 500 calories for the two fast days, so it becomes even more important to choose your calories wisely.

Alternate Day Method

This is a method where you alternate your fasting and eating periods by days and not by hours. A whole day or more goes between two eating periods. Some people fast and eat literally on alternate days. Few people also choose to eat for two days, then fast for one or two days and eat again for two days followed by fasts for one or two days. This method has been shown to work amazingly for people who follow an equally intense exercise regimen. On fasting days, one has to consume less than 25% of the caloric requirement, which comes to 500 calories or less. This method can give you up to two to four days of fasting within a week. If you consume only 500 calories or less during the fasting days, the overall caloric intake for the whole week is reduced and that is what makes this method an intense fasting method. This is a great method for efficient weight loss but definitely needs to be coupled with nutritious food choices.

Instinctive Method

This method is also known as spontaneous skipping method. This is where a person relies on their instinct to decide how and when to fast. This is more suitable for people who have chaotic or unorganized lifestyles. For someone who is too busy to pause and plan for a fast, this method is ideal. Here a person randomly decides they might fast by skipping a meal, or fast for a stretch of hours, all based on how they feel in the moment. It is like listening to their bodies and letting the body decide when and how much to fast. If according to you, for example, you feel like you can skip your lunch and wait until dinner, then by all means you do so. The next day, might not necessarily be the same. The fasting hours can differ greatly from one day to the next. This is the most flexible of all fasting types and is best for someone who is absolutely new to giving up meals for a time period. Many people are intimidated by the concept of fasts and this method helps ease them into the mindset required for fasting without making schedules and timings too taxing.

Water Fasting

This is an extreme kind of fasting technique which comes with its own bundle of risks. It requires the practitioner to stay away from food and allows only water intake. Though water fasting has been known to be very effective for weight loss, it is also thought to be risky. Most researchers and fasting practitioners are skeptical to include water fasting as one of the types of intermittent fasting. Also, it is of no given guarantee that weight lost through water fasting is not gained back once the fast ends and normal eating habits resume. Whereas such a scenario is hardly seen for intermittent fasting techniques; the weight lost is easily kept at bay with little to no effort even after normal eating habits resume, provided the food choices are healthy. Many people take water fasting to an extreme by fasting only with water for several days together, which is indeed risky. Instead this same water fasting technique can be made more compatible with the general intermittent fasting methods by allowing one such fasting day nested between normal eating days. There are no calories consumed and the practitioner relies only on water to get by. Such an approach would be more in line with what is normally followed by intermittent fasting believers.

Eat Stop Eat Method

This is a flexible way of fasting where you fast according to your needs and create your own schedule to go by. This is primarily a 24-hour period fast. One might feel the need to fast for just one day in a week. These people can have that one day nested in between normal eating days and fast on the same day next week. It is like you are eating your normal meals but stop eating for a day completely then continue normal meals from the next day onwards. For people who wish to fast for more than one day, this method gives the flexibility which is otherwise absent by following the 5/2 fasts for example. Though the number of fasts is the same, in the eat stop eat method, you are able to space out the days according to your needs and they need not be consecutive fasts as is the case in 5/2 method.

Lean Gains Method

Though this method is similar to the 14- or 16-hour fasts, it differs slightly in how practitioners go about it. Here, the goal is to fast for 14 - 16 hours coupled with rigorous workouts. This is to ensure that not only is excess fat burning but the fat is being converted to muscle directly. This happens due to the extensive physical training practitioners of this method undergo. The exercises and workout are also perfectly timed and monitored to ensure muscle buildup. It follows a strict regimen and requires quite a bit of determination and commitment. Extra care is given to what is consumed also though in general intermittent fasting does not demand it. This is to make sure that the goal of muscle and bodybuilding is achieved efficiently through foods that can help in this endeavor. This body building angle is what makes this method so popular worldwide. The fast is mostly timed to end at around noon. From the time the person wakes up until before the fast ends, this time period is dedicated to light warmups and exercises leading up to extensive workouts just before noon. Then the eating period is usually divided into two or three small mealtimes, ending in the evening, giving the person approximately 15 to 16 hours of fast.

Warrior Method

This method is very similar to the 20/4 method. Practitioners of this kind of fast are supposed to fast for twenty hours with an eating window of just four hours, but the difference here is that this is geared towards those who have extremely taxing physical activity ahead of them during the day at the time of the fast. Therefore, the meal taken is especially designed to suit their high demanding needs and is rich in proteins, fats, and carbs. It is conceptualized based on how a warrior would have time for only one large meal before beginning their day at the battlefield. This is especially helpful for seasoned intermittent fasting practitioners who have extremely busy and physically demanding schedules through the day yet would want a rigorous regime of fast.

It is important to make the right choice of intermittent fasting type. Decide what type suits you best based on your own comfort and health. Keep in mind any health concerns you may have, like diabetes, blood pressure issues, thyroid issues, or heart problems. Give consideration to your own strength and stamina, and your dedication and commitment to going without food for a considerable amount of time.

Chapter 5: The Fasting Timeline - Hour by Hour

Many people are drawn to intermittent fasting for the sole purpose of weight loss. It is a good thing, as we have been blindsided for too long by vague and complicated diet plans and exercise regimens that lead us nowhere in terms of weight loss and good health. This gets even more difficult by the fact that we have hardly any idea of what goes on in our bodies when we are following these so-called diets. But as we saw earlier, the processes occurring in our bodies are not to our advantage at all. We have also seen, in broad terms, how intermittent fasting helps us lose weight. But in this chapter let's see what actually happens in our bodies during the fast as the hours go by.

Our body, and every single cell in our body has an inherent intelligence that works toward keeping us healthy. Each cell is naturally programmed to function this way. All the healing, repair and restoration processes in our body are carried out by the help of this very inherent intelligence. But when we take a meal, the focus of the cell shifts from bettering the body conditions to digesting the partaken food. When we eat continuously for every six to eight hours, the focus is more or less always focused on digesting the meal. The body then doesn't function toward the repair and restoration purpose for which the cell intelligence was initially intended. Fasting deals with this issue. When we fast, the cell intelligence is free to concentrate its efforts on other useful processes that are necessary for cleansing and purification. As soon as the digestion of the previous meal is completed the cleansing process begins.

But even this is not as simple as it sounds. Understanding what truly occurs inside our body cells and arming ourselves with this knowledge will help us in handling our fasts better. Fasting for prolonged periods of time is not easy and having the knowledge of what is happening at the micro level will be a great motivation to carry the fasts to completion.

For the sake of this section let's consider a water fast of three days. This fast would mean that an individual partakes of a large meal and then goes without food for the next three days. What they take instead are calorie-free beverages and plain water. Creamed and sweetened coffee, or flavored water are not allowed during the fast. To derive maximum benefit from the fast, and get the best optimum results, they stick to just one large meal, full of carbs, proteins, and fibre and simply make do with plain water for the rest of the three days. Now, even though we don't generally recommend the water fast, it is useful in terms of learning what happens in the body during a fast. If you decide to partake in a water fast, like that described above, we highly recommend that you only do so under strict medical supervision.

Hour One to Hour Eight

Right from the time you have consumed the meal, your insulin levels spike. As seen earlier this spike in insulin is necessary to effectively manage the blood glucose. In these hours your body is actively undergoing metabolism. You are digesting the meal and actively producing glucose. Whatever glucose you need for your immediate activities is used up by your body cells and broken down to give you the required energy. What remains after immediate usage is converted into glycogen and stored in the cells. Think of glycogen as a readily available form of energy, that can be quickly converted into usable form. But what remains after glucose to glycogen conversion, gets packed up as fat cells. This is your body's way of saving up for the future.

By the end of the eighth hour, the insulin levels would have gone down and your body would have completed its glucose handling work by now. These first eight hours are the time, you wouldn't feel hungry at all, especially if the meal was large enough. But, if your meal was a small one, then the same process can finish in four to six hours, and you would begin to feel hunger.

By the Twelfth Hour

By the end of the twelfth hour, your body is actively producing what is known as the growth hormone. Growth hormone is a common enough hormone in kids. It is what helps our bodies grow. All our tissues, bones and muscles, grow under the influence of this one hormone. As we age, the production of growth hormone decreases considerably and stops altogether by the time we are 30 years old. This one hormone is essential to help burn fats. It builds more muscle and slows down the aging process. This is why kids have the maximum amounts of this hormone and it gradually decreases as we age because we do not need it as much anymore.

But during a fast, by the twelfth hour, our body produces growth hormone for the express purpose of helping with fat utilization. This is a vital process as this depicts that our body, understanding that no food is available turns to the easily accessible lean fat stores. This is why even those people who fast for just 12 hours see a marked difference in their weights as the process of fat burning has already begun by the twelfth hour. When you couple your 12-hour fasts with regular exercise toward the end of your fasts you have a sure recipe for success. Through regular exercise, you are increasing your body's metabolism and forcing it to work harder for providing you with the energy required for your workout.

Placing your workout strategically around the twelfth hour, will help your body burn more fats to give you sufficient energy. This will help you lose weight more effectively, even without extensive dieting or long fasts. All this would be possible only by understanding what truly happens within our cells and how we can work around these processes to turn them to our advantage.

From the Thirteenth to Fifteenth Hour

As our fast enters the thirteenth hour our body cells begin a process known as ketosis. This is the process of our cells making use of ketones for energy. Ketone bodies are produced by our liver from the breakdown of fats when glucose is not readily available. Fat burning via this process results in ketone formation and ketone breakdown releases energy. This is essential for several vital organs of our body such as the brain and kidneys to function properly in the absence of available glucose.

The higher the level of ketones in our body the more fat is being burnt. Levels of ketones are also identifiable in our blood indicating that our body is making use of the stored fats. This process kicks in around the thirteenth to fifteenth hour and goes on for about the duration of the time until glucose is again available, or until fat stores exist, whichever happens first. It is like, by the thirteenth hour the ketosis switch is switched on and it continues to actively produce ketone bodies. This is also helpful, in fact vital, for people who suffer from fatty liver syndromes. This is a common enough problem, present even in those people who are not obese, but just mildly overweight. Again, extensive diets and strenuous exercises can be surpassed through fasting. Simple elongated fasts are a simple way to dissolve these fats from the liver cells effectively.

One of the most important benefits of the ketosis process is achieving greater cognitive abilities. This is possible because our brain makes use of ketone bodies for energy and this has been shown to enhance mental clarity. Studies have shown that use of ketones instead of glucose enhances one's sharpness and brain functionality. All this could easily be achieved by a simple 16-hour fast. In these fasts, your brain would have had around three hours to process ketones and de-junk the system with the help of ketones. At this hour, your ketone level would be 0.5. This is a small yet significant amount to indicate your cells are actively producing ketones and burning fat.

By the Seventeenth Hour

By the seventeenth hour our body enters the crucial stage of repair and restoration, or "self-eating" which is popularly known as autophagy. By the seventeenth hour the autophagy process is switched on and it goes on until the time of your next meal. Fasting initiates the activation of AMPK signaling work-way that begin the process of autophagy in the cells. Through this process, the cells remove broken, dysfunctional cells, damaged proteins and the like from within it. Imagine it as the cell looking within itself for things to eat. When the body realizes that no food is forthcoming, our cells kickstart this process to look for food elsewhere. This search of food within our own cells is termed as autophagy.

Now, one might ask why if the body was looking for energy is it eating damaged and useless proteins? This is because the breakdown of these broken cells and folded useless proteins releases energy which the cells can then make use of. The breakdown process releases ATP, which the body can make use of. ATP are nothing but, Adenosine Triphosphate, which are the basic units of energy within a cell. This breakdown serves two purposes, on the one hand it is helping in the release of energy while on the other hand it is getting rid of waste proteins and dysfunctional cells which would have otherwise cost the cell extra energy consumption.

When your cells are unable to or do not kickstart the process of autophagy it gives rise to several neurodegenerative diseases. Neuro diseases such as Parkinson's disease, Alzheimer's disease etc., are all caused because of mismatched or folded proteins, which otherwise could have been prevented by the initiation of the autophagy process. This is the reason why intermittent fasting is thought to be a possible preventive measure and possibly a treatment to slow the progression of neurodegenerative diseases like Alzheimer's.

By the seventeenth hour, through the process of autophagy, your body's cells begin the process of detoxification. The seventeen-hour mark is the sweet spot for your cells to initiate a self-detoxification process. This is the reason why people widely opt for fasting techniques to initiate the detoxification process, which leaves one clearer of toxins at the end of the cleansing process.

By Twenty-Four Hours

There are several intermittent fasting techniques that have you keep a fast of 24 hours. OMAD, eat stop eat, alternate day fasting, are all techniques that help you observe a fast for a minimum of 24 hours. For people observing these fasts it is interesting as well as extremely important to know what is going on in their bodies by the end of these fasts. By twenty-four hours, there are several important functions and processes that are switched on.

Gut health is widely improved through stem cell production initiation by the twenty-four-hour mark. Your intestinal cells are frantically busy producing more stem cells, which are vital to have a healthy digestive system and efficient absorption of nutrients from your meal. It is like the body is preparing to make more use of the meal when it next comes in and is enhancing its absorption techniques accordingly. So, the next time you eat a meal at the end of your fast, your body would be more ready to digest and absorb more nutrients with greater efficiency than before, all because your body repaired its intestinal health through one 24-hour fast.

This is especially vital for people who normally suffer from poor gut health and assimilation problems. Improving gut health helps in correcting nutrient assimilative issues for such individuals by initiating stem cell productions.

Another important process that gets initiated by the 24-hour mark is the production of a chemical called BDNF. This is a brain derived neurotrophic factor. It works for the brain, how a fertilizer would work for the soil. It is produced by the initiation of the BDNF gene which gets triggered into the production process by the 24-hour mark. This chemical is essential for the survival of neurons. It plays an important role in the upkeep, growth, and production or differentiation of these nerve cells.

BDNF also causes an increase in our serotonin levels. By the 24-hour mark, a marked increase is seen in the levels of the chemical serotonin. It is an important chemical that initiates the feelings of happiness. Not just this, serotonin is responsible for regulation of mood and social behaviors. Appetite for food and good digestion are also regulated by the levels of serotonin. Sufficient and satisfying sleep and good memory retention are also handled by this one amazing chemical. All these factors can be improved by increased levels of serotonin which occurs by the 24-hour mark in the fast.

Another very important change that comes through a fast by the 24-hour mark is the decreased levels of CRP. CRP is C-reactive protein. These are treated as markers of inflammation in the body. So as the 24-hour mark nears, we see a marked decline in the CRP levels. This is vital to help heal our bodies and reduce inflammatory sites in the body. This repair can occur at injuries, wounds, intestinal or other organ linings etc., where there are chances that inflammation might occur. Another change that we can see is a decrease in blood pressure. This is especially helpful for patients with high blood pressure. For those who suffer from already decreased levels of blood pressure, you can make use of non-calorie drinks like electrolyte solutions that can help regulate blood pressure.

It is amazing how fasting for a mere 24-hour period can help regulate so many functions and processes within our bodies. Even if we do not continue our fast for more than 24 hours, we have reaped a good deal of benefits even in this short time. Few people would still like to continue to 48-hour fasts (like in the 5/2 method) or move onto 72-hour fasts like in prolonged water fasts. To know hourly breakdown of what goes on in longer fasts read on.

From 36 to 48 Hours

This is your second day of fasting and is specifically for those who are practicing a prolonged water fast. The 36-hour mark is the best time for weight loss. By this time your body is assured that no more glucose is coming in and they turn to deep stored fats for energy. These are fats that have been stored for years and these fats get burned and broken down for energy and ketone body production by the 36-hour mark. This is especially vital for people who are seen as weight loss resistant. These are people who have tried and failed at various weight loss techniques because they never reached the stage where their old and hard fats were able to burn. A 36-hour fast is extremely helpful in dealing with hard fat issues and converting them to energy.

Another change at the 48-hour mark is the exponential increase in the production of growth hormone. It is close to five times the level it was when you started your fast. This helps in preserving lean muscle and preventing fat accumulation. It has also been known to play an important role in enhancing cell and tissue longevity, healing wounds and improving cardiovascular health.

It is common to feel a little giddiness by this time. The dizzy feeling is mostly due to increased GABA levels. But, by extended fasting you experience a feeling of peace or calmness that is again thanks to elevated levels of GABA. Researchers believe that high levels of this chemical are responsible for the management of stress, anxiety and sleep issues. Neurons are continually regenerated, and this is vital for people experiencing depression and mental fog. This stage helps clear the mind and even improves memory and focus.

This second day might not be easy at all. With dizzy spells and settling feelings of lethargy and weakness, the second is decidedly tougher than the first. You might feel the need to lie down or sleep. By all means take all the rest you need so as to not over tax yourself. Remember this fasting period is for a limited time and will not and should not last longer than what is prescribed. Extensive prolonged fasting is inadvisable and can be dangerous - so, again, please make sure an extended fast is supervised by a physician.

By Fifty-Four Hours

This is the stage where insulin is at its lowest. Having low levels of insulin can be of great benefit. Very low levels of insulin ensure the continuation of the autophagy process. Your body becomes extremely insulin sensitive, which is a good thing if you are on the high-risk scale for diabetes. Lowered levels of insulin are also vital for fighting chronic diseases such as cancer and diabetes, and also reduces inflammation to a great degree.

By Seventy-Two Hours

By the 72-hour mark of the fast, your body is busy destroying old and damaged immunity cells and generating new ones. This stage is the specialist stage for heightened repair activities. Regeneration and restoration of broken or healing tissues occurs in this stage through special stem cells that reach a peak by the 72-hour mark. Be it musculoskeletal tissues, the digestive tract or any other internal organs, all are repaired through these stem cells. It is as if the 72-hour mark triggers a major overhaul of your body tissues. This is the peak of all body functions heightened to their maximum levels. After this point the functions continue for as long as the fast lasts, but might not remain at this high peak. After this stage, it is therefore entirely up to the person observing the fast to take it as far as they can. A three-day mark is the ideal, and a five- day mark is also often followed, but beyond this, it is neither advisable nor safe.

Even with regular meals between your fasts your body would still need the many micronutrients like minerals and vitamins, and other trace electrolytes through food which would otherwise go missing due to prolonged fasts. A long three-day fast once in a while is a good way to lose weight and detox your body through enhancing the rejuvenation processes in the body cells. But, again, only under medical supervision.

Understanding the hourly breakdown of the many processes that are carried out in our body during a fast is a fail proof way to stay motivated and continue our fasts with determination. Refer back to this section of the book as many times as you need to inspire yourself to take the leap and stick to your guns once you have begun your fast. It need not necessarily be a prolonged three-day fast. It can simply be a 24-hour fast which is still extremely beneficial to your body, as we just saw.

Chapter 6: Intermittent Fasting and Hormones

For women over 50 there are several hormones that come into play by this age. Some of these hormones are reduced while we age, while others are overly active. Intermittent fasting can help you regulate each of these hormones to their optimum. Let's see how each hormone gets affected or reacts through intermittent fasting techniques.

Food and Appetite Hormones

We have seen the effects of intermittent fasting on insulin and how it helps counter insulin resistance. Let's now see how intermittent fasting can help another resistance phenomenon known as the Leptin Resistance. Leptin as we know is the satiety hormone, it tells us we have had enough food and need to stop. But due to various eating disorders and hormonal changes in our body, our brain stops listening to leptin telling us to stop. Though leptin is secreted at the normal levels and is actively present in the bloodstream, our body fails to recognize that it is full and there is no further need for food.

This disorder leads to more and more consumption of food and naturally leads to abnormal weight gains. Intermittent fasting can help you counter leptin resistance. When you are fasting regularly, you are gaining a sense of self control and denying the twisted signals of the hunger hormone. Through continued intermittent fasting you will be able to pass up a plate of cake or your favorite chocolate ice cream without falling into the urge of taking a bite. Because your brain was refusing to listen to normal levels of leptin, your body was producing it in high amounts which still went ignored. But through intermittent fasting, you will be able to scale down your leptin levels making you highly sensitive to even small levels of this hormone. This is what will make you feel full when you have had a good meal. Eating more fiber-rich foods, and low-carb diets can be crucial in this scenario.

The hunger hormone, ghrelin also undergoes considerable changes during fasts. These changes have been known to have positive effects on dopamine levels which in turn improve concentration and cognitive abilities.

Female Reproductive Hormones

Estrogen and Progesterone are the female hormones responsible for various reproductive functions. For women who are younger and still in childbearing age, or menstruating age, intermittent fasting has varying effects. For some women intermittent fasting has been known to be great and non-inhibitory in terms of their reproductive hormones, while for other women who were too sensitive to intermittent fasting, it can also result in disturbed periods or temporary infertility. But, for women who are over the age of 50 this concern disappears as these women no longer produce much estrogen and are beyond the menstruating age. Therefore, period irregularity or infertility are no longer a concern.

A healthy brain-ovary axis is what determines the health of a woman with respect to the female hormones. For women over 50, without the concerns of disturbing these hormones, intermittent fasting helps maintain a healthy brain-ovary axis to ensure good hormone health.

Even for those who have not yet crossed menopause, intermittent fasting is not risky at all. It all comes down to how you introduce intermittent fasting to your body. Taking things slowly is essential. As your body gets accustomed to smaller fasting periods you can gradually move to longer fasts. It has been shown through research that all the hormonal irregularity occurs when you send your body into shock through fasting for longer periods suddenly. Give yourself and your body sufficient time to get acclimatized to the concept of fasting and you wouldn't need fear any hormonal imbalance due to your fasts.

Adrenal Hormones

Adrenal hormones are the hormones released by the adrenal glands. The adrenal glands are situated over the kidneys and are responsible for regulating our moods in times of stress, anxiety, and excitement. Of these hormones the most important is the stress hormone, also known as cortisol. A healthy adrenal-brain axis or the hpa axis is necessary to have regulated levels of adrenal hormones. When this balance is disturbed, cortisol levels spike up irregularly or go too low. This is observed to happen with intermittent fasting for longer durations of time. Cortisol levels may swing dangerously to either extreme, increasing the stress levels in our body. This leads to a condition that is commonly known as adrenal fatigue. Most common symptoms of adrenal fatigue are tiredness, muscle weakness, extreme nervousness, sleep issues, and digestive problems.

The HPA axis disturbance can give rise to several circadian rhythm issues. People who are already suffering from circadian rhythm problems find intermittent fasting for prolonged periods highly stressful. For these people it is highly recommended to follow the crescendo method of fasting. Taking it slowly and increasing your fasting hours gradually can be the key to have well-regulated cortisol levels so as to keep stress at bay.

Thyroid Hormones

The thyroid gland is a small butterfly shaped gland situated in the front portion of the neck just below the Adam's apple. It consists of two lobes on either side of the throat, connected by a small bridge like tissue. When thyroid function is normal, it is nearly impossible to feel your thyroid by physical examination. In conditions such as hypothyroidism and Hashimoto's, which is an autoimmune thyroid issue, very often the thyroid is easily felt.

Research has shown that intermittent fasting that included fasting hours during the night and the eating window during the day, had positive improving effects on hypothyroid problems. The thyroid gland is controlled and regulated by the body's internal biological clock which is also known as the circadian rhythm. Keeping the circadian rhythm functioning normally is essential to having normal thyroid functions. Therefore, if the fast can be so observed so as to not disturb the body's inherent biological clock, then it can work in the favor of those suffering from thyroid issues.

It was observed that when the fast was elongated beyond the 16-hour mark, the circadian rhythms were disturbed, and this affected the proper functioning of the thyroid gland in those suffering from hypothyroidism. Longer fasts of around 24 hours or more are highly inappropriate for patients with dysfunctional thyroid activity. Therefore, for hypothyroid patients it is advisable that they fast only for 14 to 16 hours and make it a point to have their eating window during the day. This will help balance their thyroid functioning and regulate their already irregular thyroid hormone levels.

Chapter 7: How to Implement Intermittent Fasting

We have seen what intermittent fasting is in detail. We have also seen the many pros and cons to it, its various types, and what truly happens within your bodies as you fast. But, how do we actually go about the fast? In this chapter, we will see how to do intermittent fasting, what practices to avoid and what to embrace, and what are the steps that one must take to ensure they have a successful fast.

Getting Started

Start your fast with a slow fasting schedule. Begin with a 12/12 fast or 14/12 fast at the most. Let your body get used to the fasting concept before taking a plunge into deeper, more intense fasts.

- Begin by choosing a style of intermittent fasting that you feel suits you best and that you are confident you can carry through.

- Start your fast the previous night to ensure you have a safe start to your fast while you sleep. For example, if on the night before your fasting day, you have a good large meal at 8 pm, start your fast time after two hours from your meal. So you would start your fast at around 10pm.

- For our example let's assume you are fasting the 12 to 14-hour fast schedule. If you wake up in the morning at around 6 am, you have already completed more than half of the fast. You have only four to six more hours to go to complete your fast.

- If you can engage yourself in light exercise or walking, or a bit of yoga, that could easily knock another hour off of your fast.

- Get by with water or plain or herbal tea without sugar or cream.

- By 10 am you will have successfully completed a 12hour fast and you would only need two more hours if a 14-hour fast was your plan. If 12 hours was your plan, then you can pat yourself on the back for an easy breeze through fast.

Help Yourself and Keep Motivated

To stay in the game and see yourself through to the end of your fast can be a challenge at the beginning. Extreme hunger pangs, headache, and stomach aches can make it difficult as you start your fasts to keep going hour by hour. Use the following tips to keep ahead of your fasts, avoid weakness, and stay motivated.

- Begin by keeping a journal of your fasting experience. Note everything you go through during your fast with dates. Include your fasting schedule, your eating window hours, what you had in your meal, and what you intend to have during your fast.
- Also include any symptoms you might notice. Do you feel dizzy and woozy? Write that down. Are you feeling heartburn or stomach cramps? Note that down too, along

with time. This will help you analyze your body's responses to the fast when you have everything written before you for easier comparisons. It will help you understand how many hours of the fast were symptom-free and what symptoms began after how many hours.

What to Drink While Fasting

Water

As simple as it sounds, water is one of the most important elements in our diet. While intermittent fasting of any kind does not inhibit water intake, yet people have been known to suffer from dehydration. This is mostly because we are used to drinking water following a meal or a snack. When the eatables are removed from the equation so is the water. Therefore, make it a point to drink sufficient amounts of water throughout your fast so as to not feel dehydrated.

Lemon Water

This is ideal for those who are unable to stomach drinking plain water while hungry. It is often difficult to sustain only water on an empty stomach. In such cases, you can take at least a glass of lemon water a day during your fast. Lemon water is nothing but water enhanced by adding slices of lemon in it and allowed to sit for at least half an hour. You could even add a couple of mint leaves if you feel like it. A glass of plain sugarless lemon water can give you up to 5 to 6 calories which are obviously too little to break your fast. Instead, drinking lemon water can help you feel full for a longer duration of time.

Coffee and Tea

Drink calorie-free beverages. You can take unsweetened black coffee with no cream at all. A similar tea, or even a cup of herbal tea, provided it is unsweetened is just fine too. Plain electrolyte solutions that have no sweeteners (artificial or otherwise) can also be consumed during the fast, especially for beginners, so as to make the transition easier. Remember, no milk, no cream and absolutely no sugar or artificial sweeteners!

Apple Cider Vinegar

This is a very low-calorie drink; the primary ingredient in apple cider vinegar or any vinegar for that matter is acetic acid. A tablespoon of apple cider vinegar would give you approximately 2 to 3 calories. Take a glass of plain water and mix in a tablespoon of apple cider vinegar and drink that in installments. Drinking this has shown to help burn fats and improve metabolism. Therefore, feel free to drink apple cider vinegar without the worry of breaking your fast.

Bone Broth

This is an extremely important and popular drink during the fast. People have begun to realize what a true treasure trove drinking bone broth is. It is known to help you in digestion, give you better glowing skin, healthier hair and better-looking nails too! All this because it contains collagen and is extremely beneficial when coupled with a fasting diet.

Do not make the mistake of purchasing store bought broth cubes or packaged bone broth. It is an extremely cheap and easy recipe to make while being extremely nutritious. Look through the recipe section of this book to find an easy recipe so that you can enjoy a warm bowl of bone soup!

Drinks to Stay Away From

While you would stay away from any and all kinds of solids for the duration of the fast, as obviously all solids would contain calories and sugars of their own, it is the drinks and the liquid diet that actually stumps us. So, here is a list of a few drinks that you must stay away from at all costs.

Stevia

While many intermittent fasting practitioners will tell you that it is perfectly fine to indulge in a little stevia, we think that is best left alone. Store bought stevia is a big "no" as it tends to contain glucose. Even otherwise, natural herbal-based stevia, while hailed as being calorie free is not entirely so. Instead, its sweet taste can leave you craving for more, increasing your hunger. This is not what you'd want. It is shown to have a few positive effects on cholesterol in the body, yet it is a risky trap you would walk into by consuming it.

Almond Milk

This again is a point of contention amongst many intermittent fasters. While many believe it doesn't break your fast as it isn't like true milk at all, yet I would like to believe it has sufficient calories in it to risk breaking your fast. Almonds are high in fats and other minerals. It is a completely healthy choice to make while not fasting, but not during a fast as you would undoubtedly be breaking it by indulging in this little almond goodness.

Alcohol

This is one item on the list that has a universal unanimous no from all intermittent fasting practitioners. If you are looking to lose weight and bring your body on a healthy track, alcohol of any kind in any quantity must be avoided. The point of fasting is to encourage weight loss and cleansing of the body, and drinking alcohol defeats the purpose.

Drinking it on an empty stomach has been shown to give people severe hangovers with increased intoxication of body tissues as alcohol gets absorbed into the bloodstream with a lot of ease when taken during fasts. Also, it contains a lot of calories which can easily break your fast.

Sodas

Sodas of any and every kind must be avoided. Sugar-free diet sodas are also a big "no."

Juices, Shakes and Smoothies

Fruit juices, milk shakes and smoothies are a perfectly fine addition to any meal but not so during the fast. Make it a point to include them in your feeding window if you wish but stay away from these during the fasting hours. Even juices without added sugar have a good amount of sugar in them from the fruit used. Avoid these at all costs while fasting.

Mistakes and Side Effects to Avoid

One of the biggest mistakes a person can make is to jump into a highly demanding and intense fast right from the go. In our excitement and enthusiasm to hit the weight loss goal sooner, we often make unwise choices that can harm us more. It is important to realize that there is no magic trick for weight loss. If you have accumulated pounds of fat in years, you cannot expect them all to simply fall off you in a few days. That would be inadvisable and dangerous. Give yourself at least a few weeks to a couple of months to lose weight of any significance. The slower you take it the longer it shall last. Opting for a fasting schedule like OMAD, or alternate day fasts can burn you too quickly. It will become too much to handle and you would eventually give up fasting for good. Avoid this grave mistake by going slow and choosing a simple 12/12 plan and adjusting your fasting hours to coincide with your sleeping hours.

Even when people are starting slow with smaller fasting periods, they make it difficult on themselves by undereating during the eating window. In our over enthusiasm to do things right, we often end up hurting ourselves. Undereating can potentially ruin your hormone balance after a prolonged fast. You wouldn't be able to make use of your digestive hormones to the maximum and utilize the digested nutrients to your advantage. Make good healthy quality food choices to eat during your feeding hours. Eat a good amount that you would normally eat. There is absolutely no need to under eat in your feeding hours to push the weight loss process further. Your fasting hours are doing the needful for you in that regard. Use your feeding periods to fill up on nutrients and much needed energy. Make sure to include enough vegetables in your healthy meal after a fast.

Another common mistake that people tend to make is to treat their feeding windows as times of feasting. Just because you have fasted doesn't mean you can now feast. A high calorie meal with heavy food would only negate all the effort your body just put in during the fast. Avoid greasy high-carb meals. Say "no" to junk food at all costs. You need to include not just healthy carbohydrates, fats and proteins in your diet but also look for sources of minerals, vitamins and other important micronutrients.

Some people who fast for say 16 to 18 hours a day tend to eat continuously for the remaining 8 to 6 hours. They tend to binge eat and snack on different things to keep themselves going and to make up for the lost time. This is simply wrong on so many levels. Avoid taking too many smaller meals or too many snack munches in your eating window. A good three to four eating episodes broken down to cover the 8 hours is good enough.

You might experience low blood sugar if you are not yet habituated to fasting. Pay attention to this and note it down in your journal. You can compare and analyze what foods you had in your pre-fast meal that were insufficient to last you through the 12 or 14 hours of fast. Meanwhile you can drink unsweetened electrolyte solutions to help you regain your balance and avoid feeling dizzy.

Another mistake people often make is to follow the clock too much. For example, if you had planned on a 16 hour fast and find yourself extremely tired, dizzy or too worn out to continue after about 14 hours, it is simply wise to break your fast and look at it logically. See your journal entries for the day and analyze what must have caused such heightened weakness and what you can do differently the next time. But simply sticking to the clock rigidly would be of no benefit to you, in fact you might do yourself more harm than you realize. Learn to listen to your body and much as you would want your body to listen to you.

When and How to Break Your Fast

Breaking your fast at the right time with the right food is just as important as the fast itself. Let's look at the most appropriate time and food to break our fasts with.

The When

It has been known that breaking a fast after prolonged periods of more than 24 hours, or even 16 to 18 hours for beginners, can tend to bring about a drop in energy levels after the fast breaking meal. This can be because your body energy is rushed to the digestive tract to take care of the food digestion process after a long fast and this causes the rest of your body to feel weak. You might even experience cold sweats or shivering in your limbs on breaking a fast. Therefore, it is better to have your fast broken when you are at home. Remember, we want your eating window to be in your active time of the day. So, if you tend to go to your workplace at 9 am, break your fast at 8 am so your body has time to adjust to getting food again. You can have your 8-hour window run up until 4 pm, when you can take a large meal and begin your fast. This way your toughest fasting hours that would come around eight hours after your meal can coincide with your sleeping hours, and you can break your fast just a little while after you wake up in the morning.

Learn to adapt and adjust your fasting and eating windows according to your body needs. Experiment with times during your off days so you can confidently take the plan over to your weekdays too. Like I said, work with your body and make up your own plan as you go. What might work for one might not necessarily work for you. Draft up a fasting timetable and stick with it all through one week to help you decide if it would work for you or not. You can change it up later in the next week if you feel your timing is off and not compatible with your body's needs.

The How

Just as it is important to fast slowly with workable fasting times, it is equally important to break your fast just as slowly. Do not overload yourself with heavy food. Include plenty of fiber-rich food and high protein in your breakfast. Start with a fresh fruit juice, boiled whites of eggs, and nuts such as almonds and walnuts. Fiber-rich foods like whole grains, oats, seeds like flax seeds, chia seeds etc., can all be incorporated in your meal. Try and include fish and chicken in the meal, provided they are cooked without a lot of oil and unhealthy fats. Make it a point to include healthy leafy greens like lettuce or spinach, kale and other herbs into your diet. Take things slowly. Once you have broken your fast with simple juices or salads, you can eat about an hour later, with a low carb and high protein meal.

Chapter 8: Intermittent Fasting and Exercise

People have long held onto the idea of physical training and exercise to build muscle and lose weight. Physical exertion is a vital component in your lifestyle for toning your body. We all know how important general exercise and 'moving about' is for good health. But how does one combine intermittent fasting with exercise? Is there even a need to exercise while intermittent fasting to lose weight? What if we want to build muscle while fasting, would that require exercise? We shall look to answer these and many similar questions in this chapter.

Is Exercise Necessary?

The way intermittent fasting is planned out and implemented, one wouldn't need any exercise while doing intermittent fasting for the express purpose of losing weight. Burning your fat and getting rid of excess weight is quite aptly handled by the intermittent fasting regimen itself. You do not require heavy or strenuous exercise to speed up the process. If weight loss is your only goal then intermittent fasting can safely be done without any extra physical exertion on yourself. Also, after the age of 50, exercise can become quite difficult. Our muscle and bone health is not the same anymore, we might have older troublesome injuries and wounds hindering our movements and our desire to workout. There is no need to worry in such a case, as intermittent fasting alone handles the job perfectly well.

But, if muscle gain and bodybuilding is your goal then you might want to indulge in light to moderately heavy exercise. You would need to choose a fasting type that works best for your body keeping your exercising schedules in mind. People who wish to fast as well as exercise do well with the leans gain method.

When to Exercise?

The timing of your exercise or workout regimen is just as important as the exercise itself. You do not want to over tax yourself, nor do you want to let your exercise go to waste without deriving the maximum benefit out of it. There are three approaches to timing your workouts with respect to your fasting schedules. These are before your eating window, during your eating window and after your eating window. Exercising absolutely in the middle of the fasts has a unanimous no from several health and fitness experts around the world. You would be doing yourself more harm than good by exercising right in the middle of your fast, that is to say, fasting, exercising and then continuing to fast. We shall see the other three acceptable times of exercise one by one.

Before the Eating Window

This is best suited for those who wish to build muscle and have physical training in their schedules regularly. These are people who are used to lifting weights and bodybuilding exercises on a normal basis. They do best when they follow a leans gain method. Following this method gives the practitioner a chance to fill up on much needed proteins necessary for bodybuilding as soon as the workout ends. This is why this method has gained so much popularity because it has worked so well with so many people around the world who wish to build muscle.

During the Eating Window

This is for people who are looking for better body performance and tissue recovery. Also, many people tend to feel incapable of exercising before the window as their energy levels are too low. They work best while having the option to eat while they exercise. Also, for most people, exercising while intermittent fasting is ideal during the eating window as the nutrition levels are maximum at this stage and the body is able to readily utilize glucose needed for workouts. This is truer for people who might fast for extremely long periods of time.

After the Eating Window

This is best for people who wish to exercise while they still have energy resources within their bodies at their disposal. These are people who like to have energy backups while they workout but could not fit their workout schedules in the eating windows for some reason. These are timed so as to not be too far away from the end of the eating window. This is to ensure that the body still has stored glycogen reserves available for use during the workout. If all the glycogen is used up before the workout, then it will be a strain on the body so early in the fast and it will not be advisable. Immediately after the end of the eating window is a good time for such workouts.

What Kind of Exercise is Best?

Each individual is different and has different needs. What works for one might not work for another at all. Therefore, there cannot be a common general rule for all to follow in terms of what exercise form to choose from. Still, there are few common exercise forms that almost anyone can do. We shall look at these and more in this section.

Walking

Walking is something almost anyone can do. Whether you are building muscle or simply looking to lose weight, simple yet regular walking can do wonders to your body. When this simple yet efficient form of exercise is coupled with intermittent fasting, its benefits increase by multiple folds. Though this is suitable for people of any and every age, this is the best option for those who cannot participate in other rigorous exercise regimens and need to take things slowly. Brisk walking is a great way to burn those fats without exerting yourself too much. It has been known to be great for the heart and oxidation of fat cells too.

Running and Jogging

This is again a simple exercise that is not very taxing and almost anyone can do provided no injuries hinder them. One thing to keep in mind though is to time your runs and your jogs appropriately so as to not burden your body too much. Make it a point to keep yourself well hydrated. Carry a bottle of water along with you as you go for your run. One good way to ensure your electrolytes are well balanced is to drink coconut water. As it is low in calories and full of electrolytes it would be a good way to stay hydrated during exercise.

Cardio

Light cardio exercises are best during a fast. You do not want to overtax your body and therefore must stay away from high intensity interval training

(HIIT). Fasted cardio is quickly becoming a trend and has been known to have several benefits. It is simply cardio done in a fasted state. It is done at a time when your body is no longer digesting any carbs and storing glucose. It helps in lipolysis, which is the breakdown of fats, along with fat oxidation and lowered levels of insulin.

Weight Training

This is the best option for those looking to gain muscle and also lose weight at the same time. Light weight training is a good way to burn those fats during a fast. When you workout just before your eating window you have the best chance to burn those long stored fats as your body has run out of ready glucose or even stored glycogen to fuel the exercise. You also have the advantage of refilling your energy reserves at the end of your workouts by strategically placing them before the eating window.

For those who are looking to body build, heavy weight lifting is a valid option as long as sufficient care is taken of the body during and after the workout. Primarily, time these heavy workouts during the eating window as you want your body to have proteins readily available for muscle regeneration at the end.

With intermittent fasting, though exercise isn't necessary, it is always a good thing to strain yourself a little physically. As we age, our muscle strength decreases gradually and we continue to multiply our fat stores. Indulging in light to moderate exercises along with our fasts can help us tremendously. Experts worldwide say, we need to make it a habit to "move more." Doing so will aid us in getting rid of muscle lethargy, increasing metabolism, increasing muscle strength and ultimately helping us burn fat. Make it a point to include as little or as much physical training or exercise as you can in your intermittent fasting schedules to make the most of it. You will only be heading toward a better and healthier version of yourself by exercising at least a little regularly.

Chapter 9: What Foods Should You Be Eating

In this chapter we shall see what the ideal foods are to incorporate into your intermittent fasting meal. You do not need extensive and elaborate meal planning to practice intermittent fasting and that is one of the best parts about observing intermittent fasts. But it is also true that your food choices still need to be healthy and best suited for what you have in mind. Though the focus here is on when you eat and not on what, you would still want to make wise informed choices. Whether you wish to simply remain fit and have a healthy lifestyle or to shed those extra pounds and last longer in that state, better food choices will only make your intermittent fasting journey that much easier.

Understanding Macro and Micronutrients

Macronutrients are nutrients that our body needs in large amounts for good growth and development of our body tissues. Be it muscle or bone tissues, any repair we need within our body cells, or regeneration of new cells, all require huge amounts of energy intake. These are taken care of through macronutrients. These are nutrients like carbohydrates, proteins and fats. What food you eat and what is the composition of your macronutrients decides how hungry you can get or how full you may feel. It also plays a vital role and influences your base metabolic rate, your brain functioning, and hormonal responses in your body.

Whereas, micronutrients are nutrients that your body needs in really small quantities like vitamins and minerals. Vitamins help improve immunity, skin health, and are vital for the production of energy. Minerals are important for several important processes like bone health and effective balance of body fluids.

Macronutrient Split

Studies have shown that counting calories is not always the ideal way to counter weight gain. People try to restrict calories in order to encourage weight loss. It is by the belief that restricting calories will naturally lead to a leaner body. But that is a false belief. What matters more is where those calories are coming from.

Consider 100 calories gained from eating a vegetable salad and another 100 calories gained from eating doughnuts. Though the number of calories is the same, the source is different and they each affect our body's health and functions differently. A calorie, in the end, is nothing but a measure of energy needed by our body for a number of functions. It is calculated to be about 4.2 joules of energy, regardless of the source the energy comes from. Therefore, what is needed is to monitor what type of food is contributing to the required number of daily calories, only then can we truly counter weight gain and achieve optimal health.

Now, to extrapolate our above example, to get those 100 calories of energy from salad, we would need to eat about two large bowls of a mixed vegetable salad. The same 100 calories can be had from just eating half a doughnut. The salad has the added benefit of giving us a good large dose of fiber too. Imagine yourself eating two large bowls of salad. Not only would it take you more time and effort through chewing, but the fiber from all the vegetables would leave you feeling fuller for a really long time. Not to mention how easy it would be on your digestive system. Compare this to the half doughnut. In reality, there is no comparison at all. You are nowhere close to feeling full, in fact chances are you would more likely go ahead and eat the remaining half too.

You see now why looking at the source of the calories and not just the number of them is even more important. All the major diet plans in the world work around the number of calories consumed per day. There are books and articles filled with how low-calorie diet is the thing to aim for and there are specific plans geared toward achieving a limited number of calories, like 1200 to 1600 calorie diet plans. While there might be a few plans that might work for some, counting calories consumed per day is the wrong approach to go about weight loss. Also, these do not present a long-term solution.

More effective is to balance calorie counting with the optimal macronutrient split. Let's take a look at that and see how it might fit into your fasting and general dietary regimen. The best macronutrient split for both weight loss and good health is as follows, and emphasizes a low carbohydrate approach:

Proteins should be 15% to 35% of your calories, healthy fats 40% to 60%, and carbohydrates 15% to 30%.

If you are aiming to build muscle too, then increase your proteins by a notch and bring down your fats a little: Proteins: 45%, Fats: 25% to 30%, and Carbs: 30%

Glycemic Index

Glycemic Index (GI) is a measure of how much carbs or more appropriately how much glucose a food contains. It is given as a number between 0 and 100. The highest being 100, given to pure form of glucose. This is to indicate how readily a food is digested, absorbed in the bloodstream, and it in turn affects the levels of insulin. Consuming foods that have low GI levels helps get your blood sugar levels in control and plays an important role in planning out suitable diets for healthy weight loss. Foods with low GI levels not only aid in weight loss but also reduce the risk of heart diseases and Type 2 diabetes, along with hypertension and high cholesterol.

Glycemic indices of food items are used to help you make wiser choices in your meal plan. But what is not considered or is probably impossible to measure up is how much of these carbohydrate containing food items you would eat and how you would eat them.

For example, let's consider pasta. It is known that pasta made even from refined grains has a low GI that is almost as good as whole wheat grains. But when pasta is cooked al dente, it has a considerably lower GI than overcooked pasta.

The GI is a good rough index to guide your food choices. While not completely relying on the GI of various foods, you can use it to help weed out unhealthy choices from your meal planning.

Here is a list of various food items with their glycemic indices:

FOOD	Glycemic Index
1. White wheat bread	75
2. Whole wheat/whole meal bread	74
3. Specialty grain bread	53

4.	Unleavened wheat bread	70
5.	Wheat roti with oil	62
6.	Chapati	52
7.	Corn tortilla	46
8.	White rice, boiled	73
9.	Brown rice, boiled	68
10.	Barley	28
11.	Barley flour	55
12.	Ragi flour	104
13.	Flax seeds	55
14.	Chia seeds	01
15.	Sweet corn	52
16.	Spaghetti, white	49
17.	Spaghetti, whole meal	48
18.	Rice noodles	53
19.	Fettucini	32
20.	Macaroni	47
21.	Mac and cheese	64
22.	Couscous	65
23.	Cornflakes	81
24.	Wheat flake biscuits	69
25.	Porridge, rolled oats	55
26.	Instant oat porridge	79

73. Potato crisps	56
74. Soft drink/soda	59
75. Rice crackers/crisps	87
76. Honey	61
77. Dry dates	61
78. Dried apples	28
79. Dried Apricots	29
80. Raisins	58
81. Prunes	37
82. Dried Peaches	34
83. Dried Plums	28
84. Figs	60
85. Cashew	22
86. Almonds	0
87. Walnuts	14
88. Avocado	16
89. Macadamia nuts	03
90. Banana cake (sugarless)	55
91. Banana cake	47
92. Pita bread	68
93. Coarse Barley bread	34
94. Kaiser roll	73
95. Vanilla wafers	77

Seven Anti-Aging Must Have Foods

Let's now look at a few special foods that can help you fight aging. These anti-aging foods are great at helping you lose weight too.

Olive Oil

Olive oil is a great ingredient to add to your meals. It works its wonders best when used as a dressing for salads and meat. It has high amounts of good monounsaturated fats. It has a good number of antioxidants and anti-inflammatory properties. Its most positive feature is how it can help prevent weight gain and obesity. It also works to prevent heart disease and strokes.

Berries

Berries of all kinds are a great addition to your meal. They are full of antioxidants and are great at regulating blood sugar levels and insulin action within our bodies. All berries are rich in fiber. They help fight inflammation and lower cholesterol levels too. They are great sources of vitamin C too. Blueberries, goji berries, raspberries, strawberries, acai berries, and bilberries are some of the great options available to include in your diet.

Walnuts

These are another great food to add into your meals. They are rich in antioxidants and are also a rich source of omega 3 fatty acids. They are good for controlling the process of ageing and also fighting certain cancers. They also improve intestinal health and help lower blood pressure.

Leafy Greens

These are awesome sources of vitamins, minerals, and fibre. They help fight blood sugar, heart issues, and blood pressure issues. Apart from being a great anti-aging food they also help fight mental decline. Spinach, kale, lettuce, cabbage, etc., are good examples of leafy greens.

Spices

Spices such as cinnamon, chili, and ginger have numerous health benefits. They are a sure bet to lowering blood sugar levels and help improve immunity along with enhancing brain function thereby providing anti-aging properties to your meal. When consumed in moderation they are good for fighting inflammation and regulating digestion.

Dark Chocolate

Yes, chocolate! It can help protect your skin from adverse conditions, like harsh sun and wind. It is full of antioxidants and improves blood flow while reducing the risk of heart diseases. It is also known to improve brain function.

Flaxseeds

These are rich in omega 3 fats and a rich source of high-quality proteins. They are a good source of dietary fiber and help reduce cholesterol. They are also known to lower blood pressure.

Chapter 10: Intermittent Fasting Recipes

Let's look at a few recipes that are good additions to your eating window meal plans, as well as helpful for overall health.

Chicken Veggie Salad

Ingredients

Cooked and sliced chicken breast - 1 cup

Chopped cherry tomatoes - ½ cup oz

Chopped red or green bell peppers - ½ cup

Chopped Lettuce - ½ cup

Olive oil as dressing

Salt and pepper to taste

Instructions

In a bowl add all the veggies and toss well. Add the sliced chicken and salt and pepper to taste. Stir it all up to incorporate. Drizzle a little olive oil over the top for a bit of flavor. Enjoy!

Servings: 2 Nutrition: Calories 254, Fats: 15.4, Carbs: 2.3, Proteins: 18.9

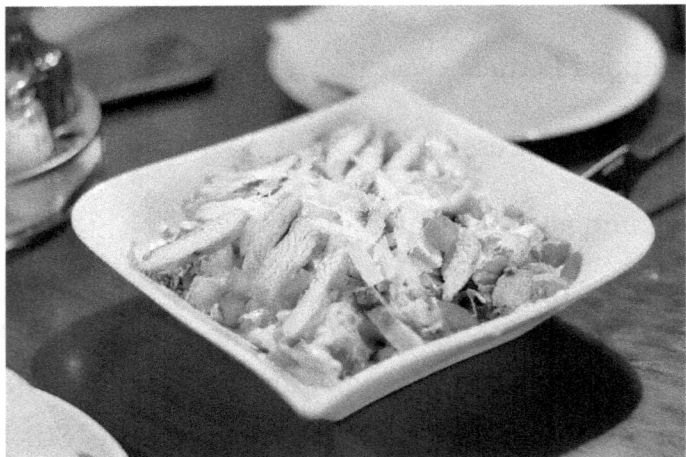

Spinach Eggs

Ingredients

Eggs, whisked - 5

Chopped red and green bell peppers - 1 cup

Baby spinach - 1 cup

Salt and pepper to taste

Olive oil - 1 tbsp

Instructions

Chop up your spinach roughly and keep aside. In a wok, add olive oil and heat lightly. Add the whisked eggs and swirl around. Fold up from the sides to help uncooked eggs coat the base of the pan again. Add the chopped spinach and sprinkle salt and pepper. Cook just until the eggs are done. Serve warm.

Servings: 4 Nutrition: Calories 112, Fats: 7.2, Carbs: 17.8, Proteins: 9.9

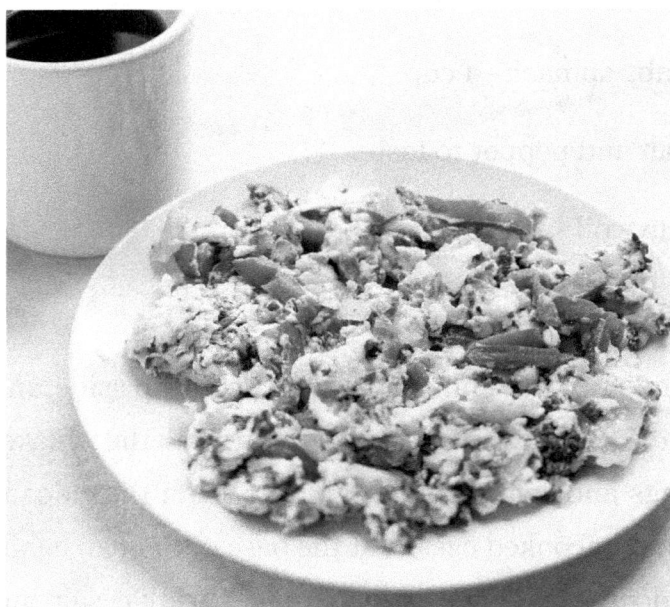

Cheesy Sausage Casserole

Ingredients

Chopped sausage - 2 cups

Grated cheddar cheese - 1 cup

Chopped Jalapeño - ¼ cup

Boiled and sliced potato - 1 large

Chopped tomatoes - 1 cup

Basil leaves - ½ cup

Cilantro for garnishing

Salt and pepper to taste

Olive oil - 1 tbsp

Instructions

Brush a casserole dish with olive oil. Line the base of the dish with the sausage slices. Cover them up with a layer of potatoes. Place a layer of jalapeños next. Cover them up with chopped tomatoes. Sprinkle salt and pepper to taste. Add the basil and cilantro over the top. Seal it all up with the cheese. Preheat the oven to 355. Bake your casserole for 25 to 30 minutes or until the top is nice and golden. Garnish with either basil or cilantro. Serve hot.

Servings: 5 Nutrition: Calories 203, Fat: 14, Carbs: 4, Proteins: 26.

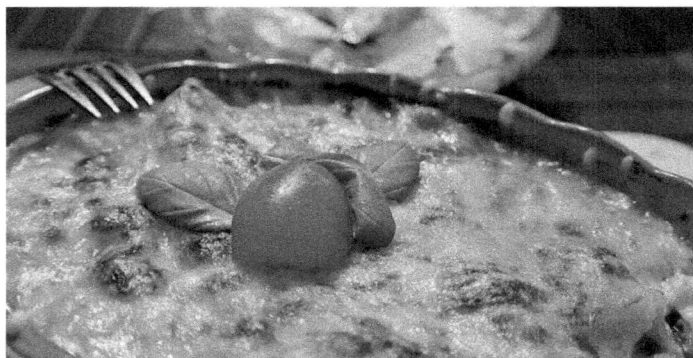

Hearty Vegetable Pasta Soup

Ingredients

Al dente cooked Pasta - 1 cup

Chopped onion - ½ cup

Peas - ½ cup

Diced carrots - ½ cup

Diced potatoes - ½ cup

Chopped garlic - 1 tsp

Vegetable stock - 2 cups or 1 cube

Salt and pepper to taste

Instructions

Coat a large heavy-bottomed vessel with cooking spray. Add in your onion and sauté for a while. When the onions turn translucent, add the garlic. When the garlic turns fragrant, add the vegetables. Stir fry a minute. Add the vegetable stock. Adjust salt and pepper to your taste. Let simmer until the veggies are done. Add in the cooked pasta and boil for two more minutes. Adjust consistency. Serve hot.

Servings: 2 Nutrition: Calories 110, fats: 0, Carbs: 24, proteins: 14

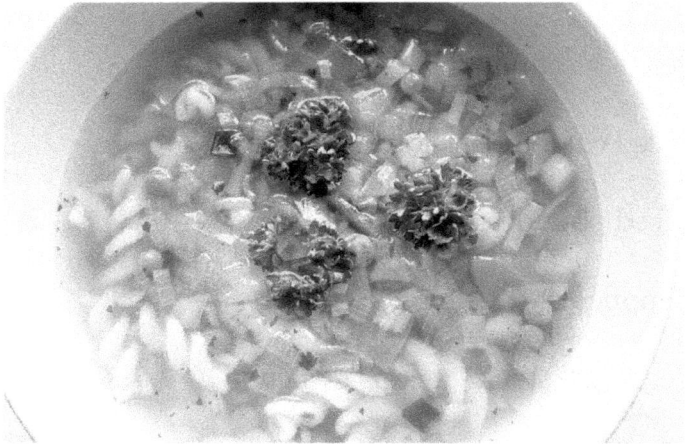

Bone Broth

Ingredients

Beef or chicken bones - 2 cups

Chopped onion - 1

Chopped carrot - ½ cup

Chopped celery - ½ cup

Chopped garlic - 2 tsp

Water - 8 cups

Onion greens to garnish- optional

Salt and pepper to taste

Instructions

In a large heavy bottomed vessel add in the bones, vegetables, and water along with salt and pepper. Bring it to a vigorous boil and let it simmer for at least 4 hours. Add the chopped garlic and simmer for 30 more minutes. Strain the broth with the help of a metal strainer to separate all the bones and veggies. Store in a glass jar in the refrigerator for up to a week or you can freeze it for later use. While reheating, adjust the water and salt according to your preference.

Servings: 4 Nutrition: Calories 35, Fats: 0.2, Carbs:2.9, Protein:4.7

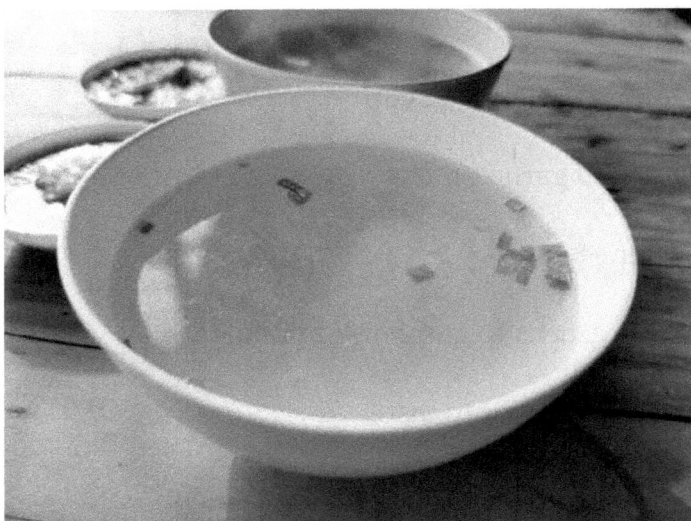

Smoked Chicken Breast

Ingredients

Chicken breast - 2

Olive oil - 1 tbsp

Red chili flakes - 1 tbsp

Mixed herbs - 1 tbsp

Salt and pepper to taste

Hot piece of whole mezquite coal - 1

Instructions

Pound your chicken with a meat mallet. Add in salt and pepper and rub well. Let sit for 30 minutes. Place the chicken breasts in a bowl, sprinkle the chili flakes, mixed herbs and olive oil. Rub it all in nicely. Brush a teaspoon of olive oil on a flat non-stick pan and add the chicken breasts. Cover and cook for 15-20 minutes flipping sides halfway. Once the chicken is done, switch off the stove. Place a small steel bowl or a piece of foil in the pan.

Place the red-hot piece of coal in it and add a drop or two over the hot coal. It will fume and smoke, immediately cover the pan with the lid and let sit for 5 minutes. Remove the foil with the coal and serve immediately. This step is to give your stove top cooked chicken a smoky grilled flavor. Enjoy warm with an accompanying salad!

Servings: 2 Nutrition: Calories 165, Fats: 6, Carbs: 12, Proteins: 28

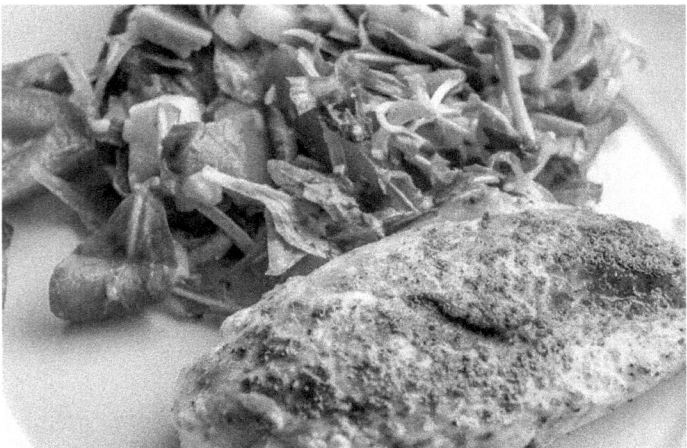

Lemon Ginger Tea

Ingredients

Peeled and grated ginger - ½ inch piece

Lemon juice - 1 tsp

Cinnamon stick - ½ inch piece (optional)

Honey - 1 tsp

Instructions

Put a vessel with around two cups of water to boil. Add the grated ginger and the cinnamon stick if using. Let it simmer for two to three minutes. Stir in the lemon juice and simmer for a minute more. Switch off the flame and strain into a cup. Stir in the honey and enjoy. If drinking during a fast, forgo the honey, it still tastes great without it too!

Servings: 1 Nutrition: Calories 20 Fats:0 Carbs:6, Proteins:0

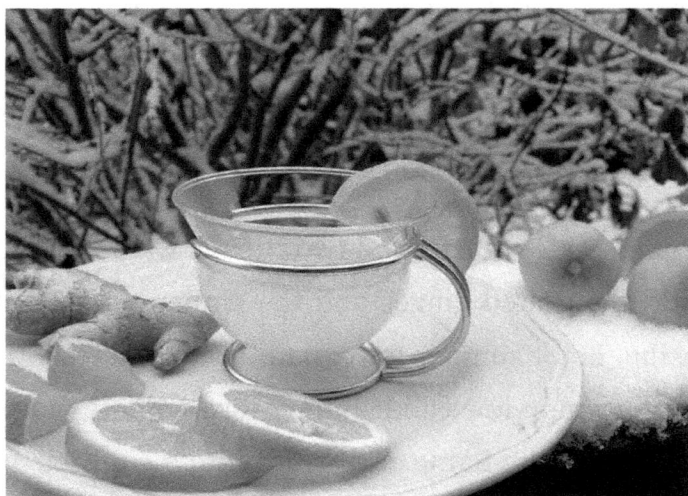

Carrot Orange Cleanser

Ingredients

Chopped carrot - 2 cups

Orange juice - 1 cup

Chopped fruit (apples/apricots/peaches) - ½ cup

Mint leaves - 1 tbsp

Grated ginger - 1 tsp

Lemon juice - 1 tbsp

Honey - 1 tsp (optional)

Water - 2 cups

Instructions

In a blender add chopped carrots, orange juice and chopped fruit of your choice. Blend until smooth. Add ginger, lemon juice, water, and honey if using, and blend some more. Use a strainer or a muslin cloth to strain the juice into glasses. Serve chilled.

Servings: 2 Nutrition: Calories 115, Fats: 0, Carbs: 30, Proteins:0.

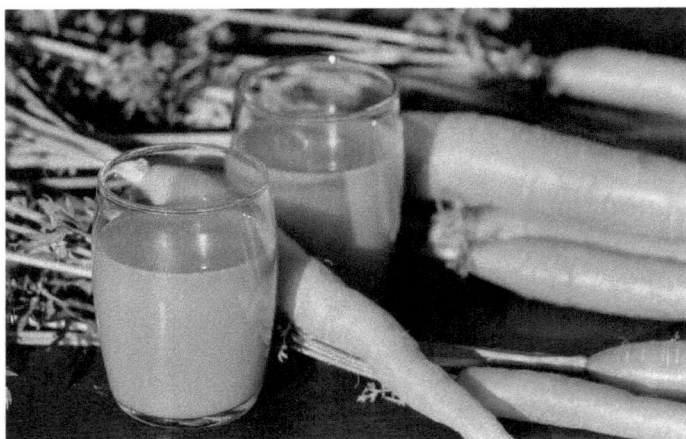

Mixed Berry Smoothie

Ingredients

Mixed Berries (raspberries, blueberries, mulberries) - 2 cups

Plain, unsweetened thick yogurt - 1 cup

Apple juice - 1 cup (or just enough for the consistency you want)

Honey - 1 tbsp (optional)

Instructions

In a blender add all the berries, apple juice, and yogurt. Blend until smooth. Adjust the consistency if thick by adding a little more juice. Taste to see if honey is required. Pour in glasses and serve chilled.

Servings: 2 Nutrition Calories: 109, Fats:0, Carbs:24, Proteins:12

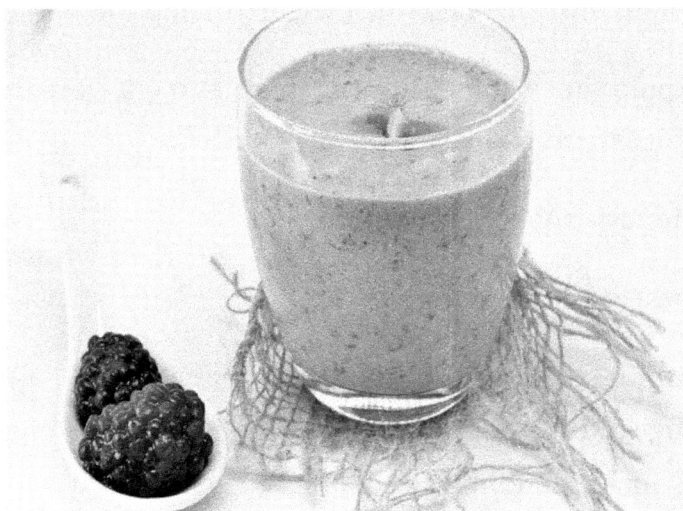

Banana Spinach Smoothie

Ingredients

Chopped banana - 1 cup

Chopped kiwi - 1 cup

Chopped spinach - 1 cup

Greek yogurt/slim milk - 1 cup

Instructions

Add all the ingredients in a blender. Blend until smooth. Pour into glasses and serve chilled.

Servings: 2 Nutrition: Calories 80, Fats:0, Carbs:24, Protein:14

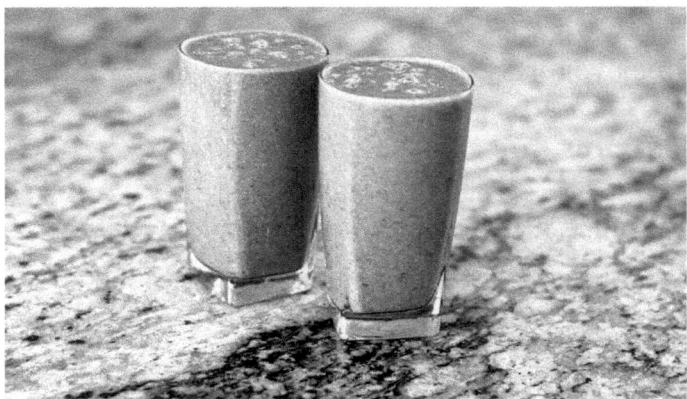

Conclusion

We are seeing a dramatic rise in diseases, infections, and deficiencies. Every year we have a new crop of fresh diseases that sends us and the whole medical world into a frenzy of searching for medicines and preventive vaccines. This wasn't the case a few decades ago. So, what changed? Why and how have we fallen this deep into this despair of sickness and ill health?

The biggest change to challenge us has been our lifestyle change. Our ancestors had neater, cleaner, and much simpler lifestyles. We, on the other hand, are plagued by depression and anxiety disorders. In terms of food, they only took on what they could eat. Obviously, lacking refrigerators, freezers, and packaged foods, they couldn't afford to buy or grow food in bulk and let it go to waste. We have every kind of food preservation and storage at our disposal. This primarily has led us to simply binge eat because we can, we eat just because we have food before us.

A major lifestyle change is the need of the day. Intermittent fasting brings you just that. It gives you a chance to bring the old-world charm of good health and lean bodies back into your lives while maintaining all the goodness of modern food practices.

Intermittent fasting isn't a new fad. Fasting has been in practice since time immemorial. People have been fasting for as long as humans have lived for various reasons. Humans have fasted for medical, spiritual, and religious reasons for years. Almost all religions have a ritual of some kind of fasting. Yet, when people are first introduced to intermittent fasting, their first feeling is that of fear. Who would want to starve? But intermittent fasting isn't something to worry about.

What we do not realize is that even without a single true fast in our lives, we still have experienced fasting. Our first day of the meal is known as 'breakfast', because we have been fasting all through the night. If you can realize this, then your intermittent fasts become much easier.

In our race toward good health and weight loss, we have passed through many doors none of which led us to our goal. Now that we know and realize what a gift intermittent fasting can be, we can hope to finally breathe in relief. Intermittent fasting when done right, can be a boon to our body.

Talk to your personal physician to get yourself a clearance nod before you proceed. Once you have that out of the way, then simply believe in yourself and take the leap into the world of fasting. If you can stay patient and committed to your goal with consistency, you can assuredly reach the peak of good health in no time at all. With its myriad benefits, intermittent fasting can be our one ticket to finally achieving our dream of losing unhealthy weight and actually maintaining it.

Before you go

I just want to quickly remind you if you haven't done so already to join my private Facebook group to have direct contact with myself and other people on the same path as you.

Just search for **Intermittent Fasting, Fuel the Brain, Lose the Fat** next time your on Facebook, answer the 3 questions provided and I'll accept your request straight away.

Also don't forget to pick up your free Intermittent Fasting cheat sheet for a quick point of reference to make sure you do things correctly from the very start.

Go to **www.thefastingfacts.com** and I will send it straight to your email.

References

Lindberg, S. (2018, October 27). How to Exercise Safely During Intermittent Fasting. Retrieved from https://www.healthline.com/health/how-to-exercise-safely-intermittent-fasting#6

Griffith, T. (2018, September 29). Fasting and Cancer: The Science Behind This Treatment Method. Retrieved from https://www.healthline.com/health/fasting-and-cancer#research

Simmons, K. (2019). Intermittent fasting for women over 50: the simplified guide to a fasting diet lifestyle for women over 50 [Mobi].

Stephens, G. (2018). Delay, don't deny: living an intermittent fasting lifestyle. Retrieved from https://www.pdfdrive.com/delay-dont-deny-living-an-intermittent-fasting-lifestyle-e176073003.html

www.ingramcontent.com/pod-product-compliance
Lightning Source LLC
Chambersburg PA
CBHW072136020426
42334CB00018B/1829